I0775031

RENAL DIET SNACKS RECIPES

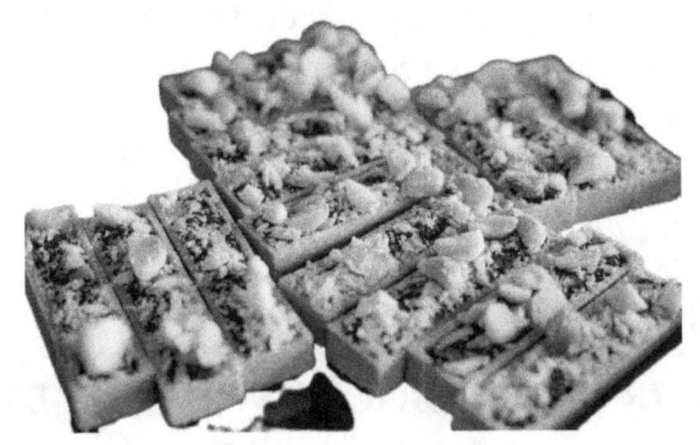

A Cookbook with Quick and Easy 50+ Meals that are Tasty, Kidney-friendly, Low in Sodium & Potassium For Optimum Kidney Health

Nancy K Doctor

All rights reserved.

No part of this publication may be reproduced, distributed, or transmitted in any form or by any means, including photocopying, recording, or other electronic or mechanical methods, without the prior written permission of the publisher, except in the case of brief quotations embodied in critical reviews and certain other noncommercial uses permitted by copyright law.

Copyright © Nancy K. Doctor, 2023.

FOR OTHER BOOKS WRITTEN BY THE AUTHOR

Scan this

TABLE OF CONTENTS

INTRODUCTION

Welcome to the realm of "Renal Diet Snacks Recipes," where the kitchen becomes an ally in your quest for renal health. This cookbook is your passport to delectable, kidney-friendly snacks that tempt the taste senses without sacrificing your well-being, whether you're navigating the complexity of renal illness or just seeking nutritional meals.

Consider your kidneys to be the unsung heroes of your body's cleanup team, working diligently to filter waste and maintain a delicate equilibrium within. However, when these key organs face obstacles, it is critical to comprehend the nature of the conflict. Kidney illness, a quiet warrior, often strikes without warning, harming millions of people worldwide.

Now, without getting into medical language, think of kidneys as the body's built-in janitors, cleaning away the debris and ensuring everything functions well. When they meet challenges, it's as if our janitors go on strike, and the entire facility becomes rather chaotic.

The Renal-Friendly Diet is your superhero costume. It's not about being deprived; it's about being empowered. Consider it a tailored handbook to assist your kidneys in their heroic responsibilities. But what exactly does this diet entail?

Consider it a milder version of the usual suspects - we've reduced the amount of certain ingredients to give your kidneys a break. Imagine your kidneys taking a deep yoga breath while you enjoy tasty, kidney-friendly food. Low sodium, low potassium, and low phosphorus are the primary actors, and we're creating a culinary symphony that keeps these components in tune.

Let's move on to the main attraction: our Renal Diet Snacks. These are more than simply munchies; they're the gastronomic equivalent of a high-five for your kidneys. But don't worry, my reader, since this trip isn't about abandoning flavor. It's all about finding a world of flavor that compliments your health goals.

Expect a smorgasbord of tastes that challenge the myth that healthy equals dull. Our snacks are a celebration of foods that respect your kidneys while also dancing on your tongue. Each recipe, from spicy dips to crispy snacks, has been created with love and nutritional expertise.

We understand that time is of the essence. These snacks aren't just good for your kidneys; they're also good companions in everyday life. Consider them gourmet pit stops - fast, healthful, and completely fulfilling.

We recognize that our readership is diverse in age, and we want everyone on board. So, whether you're 14 or 40, this handbook is for you. There's no jargon here, just clear guidance that will make you the lord of your culinary realm.

As we begin on this culinary journey together, keep in mind that the Renal Diet Snacks Recipes cookbook is more than simply a collection of recipes; it is your ally in embracing a lifestyle that honors your health while also satisfying your taste senses. Let the adventure begin!

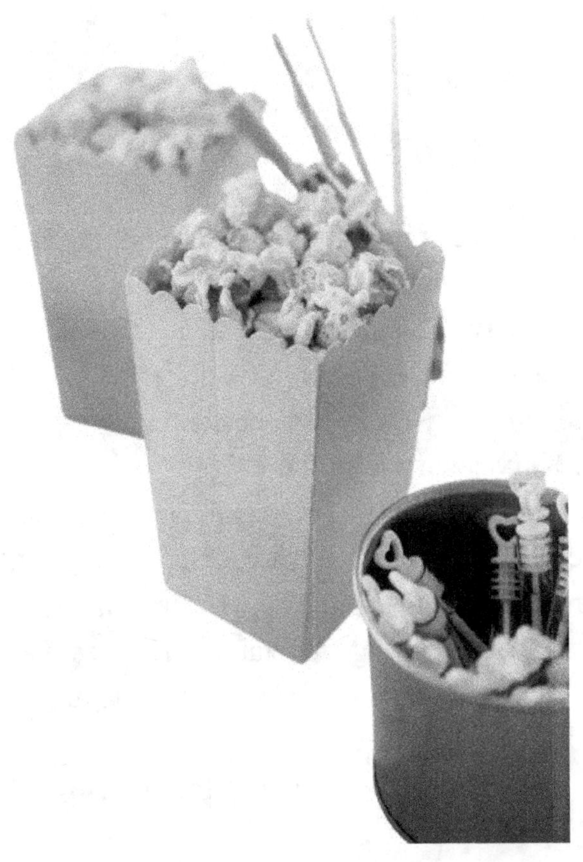

CHAPTER 1

STARTING OVER

Renal Cooking Kitchen Essentials

The correct renal cooking utensils may convert your kitchen into a haven of health and taste. Let's have a look at the key equipment and utensils that will be your constant friends in creating tasty renal diet snacks.

1. Knives with a Sharp Edge

A chef's knife is your culinary weapon, and keeping it sharp ensures that every cut is precise. A sharp knife, whether slicing fresh fruits or chopping vegetables, reduces damage to cell walls, retaining both texture and nutrition.

2. Mastering the Art of Mixing: Bowls and Whisks

Invest in a variety of mixing bowls and whisks for snacks that require a careful balance of ingredients. These techniques guarantee complete integration while preserving the integrity of renal-friendly components.

3. Temperature Control: Thermometers

Control is essential, especially when cooking proteins. A dependable meat thermometer assists in obtaining the ideal internal temperature, guaranteeing that your snacks are not only tasty but also safe to consume.

4. Measuring Cups and Spoons for Baking Precision

Precision is important in the field of renal diet snacking. Measuring cups and spoons become your best friends, ensuring that you're getting the right amount of low-sodium, low-potassium, and low-phosphorus components. This is a balanced dance, and these tools are your choreographers.

5. Baking Sheets and Pans: Oven Magic

Invest in quality baking sheets and pans for the crispy, oven-baked pleasures on your renal snack menu. With their uniform heat distribution, your products will be transformed into golden beauties without the need for unnecessary oil or salt.

6. Food Processor for Quick Chops

When speed is of the essence, your kitchen sprinter is a food processor. This tool reduces prep time for anything from cutting nuts to pureeing kidney-friendly materials, giving you more time to enjoy your culinary creations.

7. Using the Immersion Blender

An immersion blender is your secret weapon for smooth dips and creamy soups without the salt excess. It provides a velvety texture without sacrificing the nutritional value of renal-friendly ingredients.

8. Nonstick Pans That Stay Nonstick

To reduce the need for extra fats while making healthy snacks, use nonstick cookware. From sautéing vegetables to cooking lean meats, these pans ensure that your snacks are low in undesirable ingredients while being high in flavor.

Staple Ingredients

Now that your kitchen is fully equipped, let's stock the pantry with fundamental products that will serve as the foundation for flavorful and nourishing renal diet snacks.

1. Whole Grains in the Grain Game

Replace processed grains with whole grains such as quinoa, brown rice, and whole wheat. These grains provide a hearty flavor to snacks, supplying fiber and important minerals while avoiding phosphorus excess.

2. Lean Protein Sources for Protein Power

Lean protein, from chicken to fish, is the foundation of renal diet snacks. To add muscle-building deliciousness to your snacks, choose skinless poultry, fish, and plant-based proteins like beans and lentils.

3. Avocado And Olive Oil Are Good Fats.

Say goodbye to saturated fats and hello to heart-healthy alternatives. Avocado and olive oil add a velvety richness to snacks while also promoting cardiovascular health—a win-win for both taste buds and kidneys.

4. Fresh Produce with Veggie Vibrance

Consume colorful veggies such as bell peppers, spinach, and carrots. These low-potassium options provide a burst of flavor, texture, and a variety of vitamins while remaining potassium-free.

5. Fruits with Low Potassium Content

Fruits like berries, apples, and grapes will satisfy your sweet tooth while keeping your potassium levels in check. Their natural sweetness enhances snack flavor while keeping to renal diet rules.

6. Low-Phosphorus Dairy Alternatives Done Right

Choose low-phosphorus alternatives like almond milk and yogurt for snacks that require a touch of dairy. These substitutes keep the creaminess without overloading your kidneys with phosphorus.

7. Nuts and Seeds Provide A Satisfying Crunch.

Almonds, sunflower seeds, and pistachios provide a satisfying crunch to your snacks while being low in phosphorus. Sprinkle them on salads or incorporate them into granola for a nutrient-dense treat.

Cooking Techniques to Try

Let's dive into cooking techniques that transform these elements into renal diet snacks that are not only health-conscious but also a feast for the senses, now that we have the right tools and staple ingredients.

1. Grilling Excellence

Grilling is a great way to add smoky flavors to snacks without drowning them in sodium. The grill imparts a savory essence that elevates the entire snacking experience, from vegetables to lean meats.

2. Vegetables Unveiled in Steamy Elegance

The culinary ballet of steaming preserves the vibrant colors and essential nutrients of vegetables. It's a gentle method that turns greens into tender, kidney-friendly morsels that are ideal for snacking.

3. Symphony of Sautéing

Sautéing is the culinary sprint, infusing flavor into snacks in just minutes. You can make savory wonders without drowning your ingredients in sodium by using a quality nonstick pan and a touch of heart-healthy oil.

4. Oven Magic

Baking is the alchemy of turning raw ingredients into golden treats. It's the ideal method for making kidney-friendly cookies, muffins, and snacks that are both healthy and delicious.

5. Blissful Blending

Blending works wonders for dips, spreads, and creamy treats. This technique, whether using an immersion blender or a food processor, ensures a velvety texture without the need for extra fats or sodium.

Shopping Guide

As we embark on the journey of crafting delectable renal diet snacks, the first pitstop is the vibrant world of fresh produce. Consider the produce section of your playground, where each choice contributes not just to the flavor but also to the kidney-friendly essence of your snacks.

1. Colorful Bounty

When selecting vegetables, opt for a colorful array that mirrors the rainbow. Bell peppers, zucchini, and carrots are not just visually appealing; they are low in potassium, making them ideal for creating snacks that burst with flavor without compromising kidney health.

2. Leafy Greens

Leafy greens such as spinach and kale bring a nutritional powerhouse to your snacks. Rich in vitamins and minerals while being low in potassium, they elevate the health quotient of your creations without raising concerns for kidney function.

3. Fruits with Low Potassium Content

The sweetness of fruits can be a delightful addition to your snacks, but not all fruits are created equal in the renal diet. Opt for low-potassium options like berries, apples, and grapes. Their natural sweetness adds a fruity kick without tipping the potassium scale.

4. Balanced Berries

Berries, in particular, are not just low in potassium but also pack an antioxidant punch. From strawberries to blueberries, these tiny flavor bombs elevate the taste of your snacks while contributing to overall health.

5. Mindful Melons

While melons can be refreshing, it's essential to choose wisely. Watermelon and honeydew are low-potassium choices that bring a hydrating element to your snacks, perfect for those warm days when a cool treat is on the menu.

Reading Food Labels for Sodium, Potassium, and Phosphorus Content

In the intricate dance of renal diet snacks, knowledge is your partner, and food labels are the choreography that ensures harmony. Understanding how to decipher these labels is akin to holding the key to a kingdom where every snack aligns with your kidney-friendly goals.

1. Sodium Surveillance

Sodium, often sneaky in its appearance, can be unveiled through vigilant label reading. Snack foods, even those that don't taste overly salty, may hide sodium content. Opt for products labeled "low-sodium" or "sodium-free," and be cautious of high-sodium additives like monosodium glutamate (MSG).

2. Potassium Patrol

Potassium, a mineral vital for many bodily functions, needs careful monitoring in the renal diet. Scan labels for potassium content, and favor snacks with lower levels. Fresh produce is generally potassium-friendly, but packaged snacks may contain potassium additives. Be discerning, especially with processed foods.

3. Phosphorus Prowess

Phosphorus, an often overlooked player, deserves attention in the renal diet. Processed foods, carbonated drinks, and some dairy products can be high in phosphorus. Scrutinize labels for phosphorus additives, and opt for snacks with lower phosphorus content to safeguard your kidney health.

4. Serving Size Wisdom

Beyond individual nutrient content, pay heed to serving sizes. Snacks may appear kidney-friendly until you realize you've consumed multiple servings in one sitting. The serving size provides context for the nutritional information and helps you maintain portion control for optimal renal health.

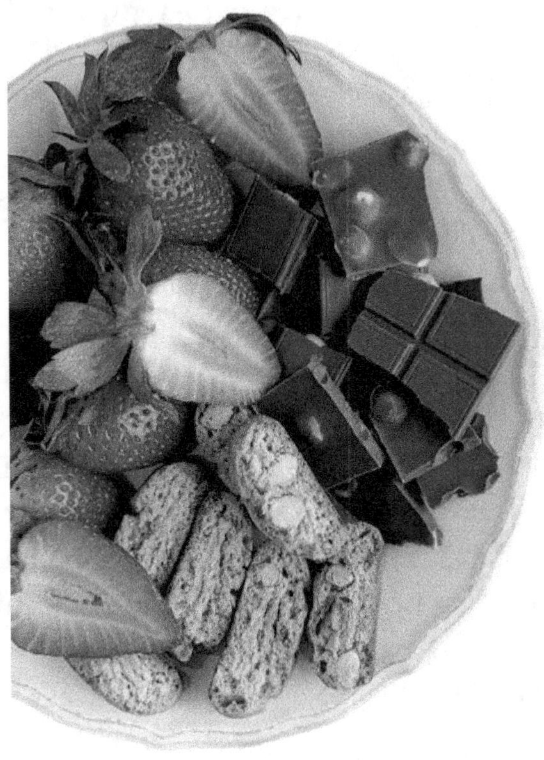

CHAPTER 2

Finding Renal-Friendly Brands

Navigating the aisles of the grocery store can be an adventure, and finding renal-friendly brands is like discovering hidden treasures. These brands understand the delicate balance required for renal snacks, offering options that cater to your dietary needs without compromising on taste.

1. Low-Sodium Champions

Certain businesses specialize in making low-sodium snacks that don't sacrifice flavor. From crackers to popcorn, research products branded "low-sodium" or seek out companies with a focus on decreasing salt levels. Your taste buds will thank you, and your kidneys will too.

2. Potassium-Conscious Choices

As knowledge rises about the significance of potassium in the diet, certain businesses are leading the charge in delivering potassium-conscious alternatives. Look for foods that emphasize reduced potassium levels, especially in goods like granola bars and packaged nuts.

3. Phosphorus-Friendly Fare:

While not as often touted, several brands realize the role of phosphorus in renal health. Explore products that consciously limit phosphorus additives, particularly in convenience snacks like pre-packaged trail mixes and energy bars.
Chapter 2: Kidney-Friendly Foods

Low-Sodium Flavor Enhancers

In the intricate dance of renal diet snacks, the flavor is the star, and mastering the art of low-sodium enhancements is the key to a culinary symphony that tantalizes the taste buds. Let's explore the world of savory notes and fragrant subtleties without sacrificing the precise balance of salt.

1. Herbs & Spices

Say goodbye to the assumption that minimal sodium implies compromising flavor. Herbs and spices are the hidden heroes of the renal kitchen, delivering a multitude of flavors without the need for excessive salt. From rosemary to cumin, each spice and herb contributes its distinct personality to your munchies, converting them into a kaleidoscope of gourmet delights.

2. Citrus Zest

When salt steps aside, orange zest jumps in. Grate the colorful peels of lemons, limes, and oranges to infuse your snacks with a blast of freshness. This not only adds a zing to the flavor but also enriches the sensory experience, opening your palette to new depths of taste.

3. Vinegar Varieties

From balsamiq to apple cider vinegar, these tangy elixirs are low-sodium companions that improve the complexity of your munchies. Drizzle them over salads or use them as a marinade for foods to impart a subtle acidity that keeps your taste receptors interested.

4. Garlic and Onion:

The powerful combo of garlic and onion, whether fresh, minced, or powdered, gives a flavorful depth to your food. They are low in sodium and rich in culinary expertise, ensuring your snacks are not simply healthful but also delightfully fragrant.

Low-Potassium Substitutes

Navigating the realm of renal diet snacks demands a thorough awareness of potassium, and developing replacements that keep flavor while sticking to dietary requirements is the next stage in this culinary adventure.

1. Applesauce Magic

In baking and cooking, where potassium-rich components may hide, applesauce steps in as a wonderful alternative. It adds sweetness, moisture, and a bit of fruity essence to your snacks without sacrificing on texture or taste.

2. Berries for Bananas

While bananas are a potassium powerhouse, berries offer a lower-potassium option for that rush of sweetness in your snacks. Whether fresh or frozen, berries provide a delicious tanginess that compliments numerous snack dishes.

3. Cauliflower Craze

Cauliflower is the chameleon of the vegetable kingdom, morphing into rice, pizza crust, or even mashed "potatoes." Its low potassium concentration makes it a flexible replacement, ensuring that your snacks are not just delicious but also potassium-conscious.

4. White Bread Wisdom:

In the area of grains, finding low-potassium bread options becomes vital. Opt for white bread over whole wheat or multigrain choices, since it tends to have lower potassium levels, ensuring your sandwiches and toast stay kidney-friendly.

Low-Phosphorus Alternatives

Phosphorus, the often-overlooked player in the renal diet, demands careful study. Let's examine options that retain the nutritious integrity of your snacks without tipping the phosphorus scale.

1. Almond Flour Alchemy

For those delighting in baking escapades, almond flour steps in as a low-phosphorus alternative to regular wheat flour. It gives a delicious nuttiness to your food, guaranteeing that your taste receptors indulge in the richness of almonds without the phosphorus excess.

2. Rice versus Beans

While beans are high in nutrients, they can also be high in phosphorus. Using rice as a snack basis provides a lower-phosphorus option, ensuring that your culinary creations are not only diversified but also considerate of your kidney health.

3. Non-Dairy Treats:

In the world of creamy pleasures, choosing non-dairy milk alternatives such as almond or rice milk is a low-phosphorus option. These alternatives keep the velvety feel without adding too much phosphorus to your food.

4. Elegance of Egg Whites

Consider using egg whites instead of whole eggs for protein-rich snacks. This straightforward substitute reduces phosphorus consumption while maintaining protein content, providing a careful balance that appeals to both taste and renal health.

Options That Are Both Tasty And Kidney-friendly

The quest for flavor takes center stage when it comes to producing renal diet snacks, and learning how to infuse your creations with flavor while sticking to kidney-safe standards is an art worth mastering.

1. Elevating Herb Infusions Without Increasing Sodium

Herbs are the culinary masters of kidney-friendly alternatives. Herbs bring a symphony of flavors without raising the sodium curtain, from the earthy notes of thyme to the refreshing kick of mint. Incorporating a variety of herbs into your snacks ensures a palate-pleasing experience while adhering to the low-sodium principles of the renal diet.

2. Citrus Symphony

Citrus fruits, with their vibrant flavors, act as conductors of a flavor symphony that delights while not jeopardizing kidney health. Citrus zest or juice gives your snacks a zing, introducing a burst of flavor without tipping the potassium scale. It's a revitalizing and kidney-friendly way to enhance the sensory experience.

3. Spice Harmony

Spices, the culinary world's magicians, add depth and warmth to your snacks without relying on sodium. Cumin, paprika, and coriander are a few examples of kidney-friendly spices that add complexity and character to your dishes. Using a variety of spices ensures that your snacks are flavorful and free of the sodium pitfalls that frequently accompany processed options.

4. Savory Delights Without Phosphorus Overload

Umami, the fifth taste frequently associated with savory richness, can be achieved without the use of high-phosphorus ingredients. Using umami-rich foods like mushrooms, tomatoes, and soy-based products adds a savory elegance to your snacks, demonstrating that kidney-safe alternatives can be just as indulgent and satisfying as their traditional counterparts.

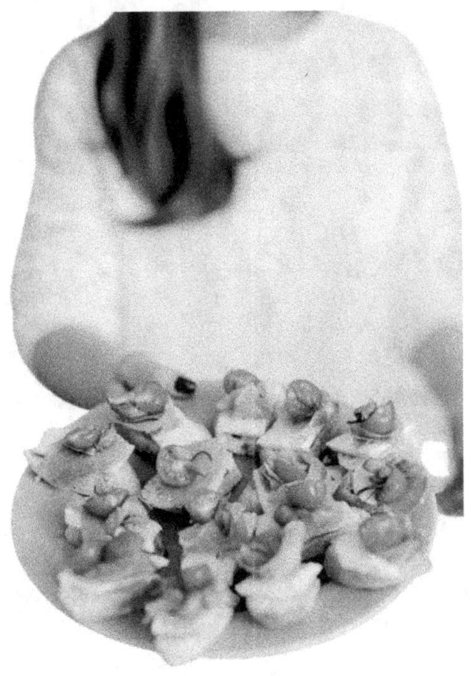

CHAPTER 3

RECIPES FOR DELICIOUS AND NUTRITIOUS SNACKS

1. Ginger Soft Cookies

Ingredients:
- 2-¼ cups white all-purpose flour
- 2 teaspoons ginger powder
- 1 tsp. baking soda
- ¾ teaspoon cinnamon powder
- ½ teaspoon clove powder
- 1 pound unsalted butter
- 1-⅛ cup
- Granulated sugar
- ¼ cup low-cholesterol liquid egg substitute
- A quarter cup of molasses

Preparation:
1. Preheat the oven to 350 degrees Fahrenheit.

2. Combine the flour, ginger, baking soda, cinnamon, and cloves in a medium mixing bowl. Place aside.
3. In a large mixing bowl, beat butter for 30 seconds on medium speed with an electric mixer. 1 cup sugar should be mixed in.
4. Beat in the liquid egg substitute and molasses.
5. Mix the flour into the egg mixture.
6. Form dough into 1-½"balls, about 1 heaping tablespoon for each.
7. Coat the balls in the remaining sugar.
8. Place the balls on an ungreased cookie sheet about 2-½" apart.
9. Bake for 10 minutes or until golden brown and puffy. (Avoid overbaking.)
10. Allow the cookies to cool for two minutes on the baking sheet before transferring them to a wire rack to finish cooling.

Tips:

- If the dough is too soft to handle, chill it for half an hour.
- To keep cookies soft, store them in a tightly sealed container.

<u>Nutritional information:</u> 142 calories, 2g protein, 21g carbohydrate, 6g fat, 16mg cholesterol, 60mg sodium, 70mg potassium, 18mg phosphorus, 13mg calcium, 0.4g fiber, 12g added sugar

2. Bars Of Granola

Ingredients:

- ¾ cup reduced-sodium peanut butter
- ¼ cup of honey
- ½ cup brown sugar, packed
- ½ cup corn syrup
- 5 tbsp butter
- 2 tsp vanilla extract
- 3⅓ cups rolled oats
- ¾ cup pretzels, unsalted
- ¼ cup semisweet chocolate chips
- Ten caramel candies

Preparation:

1. Preheat the oven to 350 degrees F.
2. In a large bowl, stir together the peanut butter, honey, butter, brown sugar, corn syrup, and vanilla until smooth.
3. Include the remaining ingredients: oats, pretzels, chocolate chips, and caramels. Stir well.

4. Gently spread the mixture into a 13 x 9-inch greased pan.
5. Bake for 20–25 minutes.
6. Allow to cool on a wire rack before slicing into bars.
7. Cut into 1 x 4½ inch bars. This recipe should create 26 bars.

Nutritional information: Calories 183cal, Carbohydrates 27.2g, Dietary Fiber 1.5g, Protein 3.5g, Fat 7.6g, Saturated Fat 2.7g, Sodium 27.2mg, Potassium 104.4mg, Calcium 21.1mg, Phosphorus 75.4mg.

3. Fruit Crisp

Ingredients:
- A twenty-one ounce can of peaches in their juice (drained)
- 1 tsp lemon juice
- ½ cup brown sugar
- ¼ cup white flour
- ¾ cup oats
- ½ tsp cinnamon
- ½ tsp nutmeg
- ¼ stick chilled butter, unsalted

Preparation:
1. Preheat the oven to 350 degrees F.

2. In a greased muffin tray, drop in peaches and sprinkle with lemon juice.
3. Combine brown sugar, flour, oats, and spices.
4. Mix in the butter until the combination looks like wet sand.
5. Sprinkle over the fruit mixture.
6. Cook/Bake for 25-30 minutes or until the top is golden and bubbling.

Nutritional information: Calories 310cal, Carbohydrates 60.9g, Dietary Fiber 3.9g, Protein 3.9g, Fat 7g, Saturated Fat 3.8g, Sodium 15.6mg, Potassium 296.1mg, Calcium 46.4mg, Phosphorus 99.8mg.

4. Baked Pita Crisps

Ingredients:
- 3 (6″) pita rounds
- 2 tbsp olive oil
- chili powder to taste

Preparation:
1. Preheat the oven to 350° F.
2. Divide each pita into two halves (resulting in six pita rounds).
3. Cut each pita into 8 wedges.

4. Coat the wedges with olive oil and season with chili powder.
5. Bake for about 15 minutes until crisp.

Nutritional info: Calories: 80 KCal, Protein: 2g, Carbohydrates: 8g, Total Fat: 4g, Sodium: 80 mg, Phosphorus: 14 mg, Potassium: 26mg.

5. Bannock (Luskinikn)

Ingredients:
- 5 cups (1250 ml) white flour
- 2 tsp (10 ml) cream of tartar
- ¾ tsp (7.5 ml) baking soda
- ½ cup (125 ml) unsalted, non-hydrogenated margarine
- 2¼ cup (310 ml) water
- One tablespoon (15 ml) of melted unsalted, non-hydrogenated margarine.

Preparation:
1. Preheat the oven to 350°F.
2. In a large basin, whisk together all the dry ingredients.
3. Make a well amid the flour and fill it with some liquid and oil or margarine. Stir it gently with a spoon or fork.
4. Continue adding liquid until the dough reaches a soft ball consistency. You

might have to add extra liquid or flour as you whisk.

5. Set aside some flour in the bowl so that you can knead the dough and shape it into a loaf pan.

6. Inside the bowl, gently knead the dough for approximately a minute.

7. Pat the dough flat into a bread pan of your preference. A 10" round cake pan was utilized.

8. Cut the bread into parts after making a cross on it. The incision is approximately 14" deep.

9. Bake for approximately 45 minutes or until the edges and top are a golden brown hue.

10. Remove from the oven. Spread margarine over the top to make it tender.

11. Cover with a clean dish towel, and let cool.

Nutritional info: Calories: 267.4KCal, Protein: 5.5g, Carbohydrates: 40.1g, Fiber: 1.6g, Total Fat: 9.1g, Sodium: 84.9mg, Phosphorus: 57.66mg, Potassium: 140.89mg.

6. Favorite Cranberry Salad

If you're yearning for something sweet and sour, look no further. This favorite cranberry salad is sure to gratify and is ideal for patients with diabetes; CKD Stage 1, 2; CKD Stage 3, 4; those on dialysis and CKD 5, and kidney transplant recipients.

Ingredients:

- 12-ounce bag of fresh cranberries
- 1 cup white sugar
- 2½ pounds red grapes, halved
- 9 ounces crushed pineapple, drained
- 2 cups mini-marshmallows
- 8-ounce tub of lite whipped topping

Preparation:

1. In a food processor, grind the cranberries to a fine texture.
2. Put the cranberries, sugar, and pineapple in a strainer and place it over a bowl.
3. Allow the mixture to drain in the refrigerator for at least 12 hours.
4. Discard the juice that drains off.
5. Add the rest of the ingredients to the cranberry mixture and stir.
6. Allow the salad to cool for a maximum of 4 hours.

7. Serve cold and enjoy!

Nutritional Information: Calories 118 cal, Carbohydrates 26.7g, Dietary Fiber 1g, Protein 0.8g, Fat 1.6g, Saturated Fat 1.3g, Sodium 15.6mg, Potassium 77.5mg, Calcium 13.7mg, Phosphorus 15.6mg.

7. Fresh Fruit Cranberry Dip

Ingredients:

- 8 oz. sour cream
- ½ cup cranberry sauce (whole berries)
- a quarter teaspoon of nutmeg
- ¼ teaspoon ginger powder
- 4 cups pineapple, fresh
- four medium apples
- four medium pears
- 1 tsp. lemon juice

Preparation:

1. In a food processor, combine the sour cream, cranberry sauce, nutmeg, and ginger until well combined. Transfer to a small bowl.
2. Cut the pineapple into bite-size chunks. Cut each apple and pear into 12 slices. To avoid browning, toss apple and pear pieces with lemon juice.

3. Arrange the fruit on a dish, with the dip bowl in the center. Refrigerate until ready to serve.

Tip:

Keep leftover dip in the refrigerator for up to 3 days.

Nutritional Info: Calories 70cal, Protein: 0g, Carbohydrates: 13g, Fat: 2g, Cholesterol: 4mg, Sodium: 8mg, Potassium: 101mg, Phosphorus: 15mg, Calcium: 17mg, Fiber: 1.5g, Sugar: 2g

8. Popcorn for a Special Day

Ingredients:
- 2 tablespoons 2% fat milk
- a quarter cup of small marshmallows
- 2 teaspoons sprinkles
- 4-ounce cake mix (golden yellow)
- 4 cup popcorn (air-popped)
- 1 tablespoon vanilla extract

Preparation:
1. Make some popcorn.
2. Take out any kernels.
3. In a saucepan over low heat, melt marshmallows, vanilla, and milk. Continuously stir.
4. Mix in the cake mix and popcorn.

5. Hands should be sprayed with nonstick cooking spray.
6. Form ½ cup of the mixture into a ball.
7. Proceed with the remaining ingredients.Place popcorn balls on waxed paper and top with sprinkles.

Nutritional information: Calories 139cal, Carbohydrates 28.9g, Dietary Fiber 1g, Protein 1.9g, Fat 1.4g, Saturated Fat 0.4g, Sodium 126mg, Potassium 1.9mg, Calcium 36.6mg, Phosphorus 85.9mg.

9. Sweet Popcorn Balls

Ingredients:

- 16 cups popped popcorn, unsalted
- 2 cups Karo® dark corn syrup
- 2 cups brown sugar
- 1 cup water
- 1 tablespoon vinegar
- 4 tablespoons whipped butter

Preparation:

1. Pop popcorn and place it in a big bowl. Set away for use later.
2. Mix syrup, brown sugar, water, and vinegar in a pot. Cook over medium heat, stirring regularly until the mixture

boils. Continue cooking and stirring virtually constantly around 15-20 minutes on medium heat. Cook to a hard ball stage (until a small quantity of mixture forms a hard ball when tested in extremely cold water.)

3. Remove from heat, rapidly add butter, and whisk.

4. Slowly pour the mixture over popped popcorn in a big bowl, while mixing well.

5. Shape into balls, applying minimal pressure.

6. Wrap each popcorn ball with plastic wrap and store it in an airtight container.

Tips:

Butter hands, or better yet, wear rubber gloves with butter on them. The popcorn won't cling as terribly and is not as hot!

Nutritional Info: Calories 241cal, Protein 1g, Carbohydrates 48g, Fat 5g, Cholesterol 3mg, Sodium 80mg, Potassium 81mg, Phosphorus 26mg, Calcium 15mg, Fiber 1.0g.

10. Sweet & Sour Meatballs

Ingredients:
- 1 pound ground turkey, 7% fat
- 1 big egg
- ¼ cup unseasoned bread crumbs
- 2 tablespoons onion
- 1 teaspoon garlic powder
- ½ teaspoon black pepper
- ¼ cup canola oil
- 6 oz. grape jelly
- ¼ cup bottled Heinz® chili sauce

Preparation:
1. Blend the ground turkey, egg, bread crumbs, finely diced onion, garlic powder, and pepper.
2. To create 48 meatballs, shape the turkey mixture into ¾ -inch balls.
3. Heat the oil in a large pan over medium heat and cook the meatballs. Turn several times to ensure uniform browning. Cook until the meatballs are completely cooked through.
4. In a microwave-safe dish, combine the jelly and chili sauce and heat for 1 to 2 minutes, or until the jelly is liquefied. Pour over the meatballs in a chafing dish

or slow cooker set on low heat, stirring well.

Tips:

- This recipe works best with 7% fat ground turkey. Ground turkey breast meat meatballs are not as moist.
- Ground beef or pig can be used in place of ground turkey.

Nutritional Info: Calories: 127cal, Protein: 9g, Carbohydrates: 14g, Fat: 4g, Cholesterol: 41mg, Sodium: 129mg, Potassium: 148mg, Phosphorus: 89mg, Calcium: 15mg, Fiber: 0.2g.

11. Soup with Sour Cherries from Hungary

Ingredients:

- 1-½ cup fresh cherries
- 3 cups water
- ⅓ cup sugar
- ⅛ teaspoon salt
- 1 tablespoon all-purpose white flour
- ½ cup reduced-fat sour cream

Preparation:

1. Remove pits from cherries.

2. Add water to a medium saucepan combined with cherries, sugar, and salt. Bring to a boil then simmer at a very low heat for 10 minutes.
3. Remove 2 tablespoons of liquid and put aside for garnish.
4. Remove another ¼ cup of the liquid and allow it to cool somewhat.
5. Whisk together with the flour and sour cream then return to the saucepan.
6. Simmer for another 5 minutes over low heat.
7. Remove from heat and allow to cool.
8. Serve in a soup dish. As a garnish, swirl in the saved cherry juice.

Tips:

- Adjust the sugar or Splenda to your liking.
- When Splenda or another sugar substitute is used in place of sugar, the carbohydrate content is 16 grams per serving, which equals one Carbohydrate Choice.
- To make this dish even easier, look for canned cherries in juice or light syrup.

Nutritional Info: Calories: 144cal; Protein: 2g; Carbohydrates: 25g; Fat: 4g; Cholesterol:

12mg; Sodium: 57mg; Potassium: 144mg; Phosphorus: 40mg; Calcium: 47mg; Fiber: 1.0g.

12. Sour Cream with Cucumbers

Ingredients:
- 2 cucumbers, medium
- a quarter teaspoon of salt
- 1 large sweet onion
- 1 tablespoon white wine vinegar
- 1 teaspoon of canola oil
- ⅛ teaspoon ground black pepper
- ½ cup low-fat sour cream

Preparation:
1. Cucumbers, peeled and thinly sliced, should be placed in a medium-sized serving bowl.
2. Season with salt. Allow for 15 minutes before rinsing and pressing away extra moisture.
3. Slice the onion thinly.
4. Toss the cucumbers with the other ingredients.
5. Before serving, chill in the refrigerator.

Tips:

- This is an excellent complement to any meal, but particularly to beef and hog meals.
- Instead of using two regular cucumbers, use one large "English hothouse" seedless cucumber.
- If you don't want to use the onion, the cucumbers are still delicious.

Nutritional Info: Calories: 64, Protein: 1g, Carbohydrates: 4g, Fat: 5g, Cholesterol: 3mg, Sodium: 72mg, Potassium: 113mg, Phosphorus: 24mg, Calcium: 21mg, Fiber: 0.8g, Sugar: 0g.

13. Tortilla Chips with Sweet and Spicy Sauce

Ingredients:

- ¼ cup melted butter
- 1 tsp. brown sugar
- ½ teaspoon chile powder, ground
- a half teaspoon of garlic powder
- ½ teaspoon cumin powder
- ¼ teaspoon cayenne pepper, ground
- 6 flour tortillas, 6" in diameter

Preparation:

1. Preheat the oven to 425 degrees Fahrenheit.
2. Spray a baking sheet with nonstick cooking spray.
3. In a separate bowl, mix together melted butter, brown sugar, and spices.
4. Cut each tortilla into 8 wedges and arrange on a baking sheet in a single layer.
5. Coat tortillas with seasoning mixture using a pastry brush.
6. Bake for 8 minutes, or until golden brown, and serve warm or cold.
7. Extra chips should be stored in an airtight container.

Tips:

- To easily cut tortillas into wedges, use kitchen shears.
- Corn tortillas can be used in place of flour tortillas for a lower sodium snack (48 mg), but the phosphorus content is higher (63 mg).

Nutritional Info; Calories: 115, Protein: 2g, Carbohydrates: 11g, Fat: 7g, Cholesterol: 15mg, Sodium: 156mg, Potassium: 42mg, Phosphorus:

44mg, Calcium: 31mg, Fiber: 0.6g, Added Sugar: 1g.

14. Snack Mix with Spicy Crunch and Munch

Ingredients:
- 4 cups Rice Chex® Ralston Purina® cereal
- 2 cups Crispex® cereal from Kellogg's
- 3 cups small oyster crackers
- 1 cup pretzel twists, unsalted
- 5 tbsp trans fat-free unsalted margarine
- 1 teaspoon of chili powder
- ¼ teaspoon cumin powder
- a half teaspoon of garlic powder
- a quarter teaspoon of cayenne pepper
- 1 tablespoon Worcestershire sauce
- 1 teaspoon lemon juice

Preparation:
1. Preheat the oven to 250 degrees Fahrenheit.
2. In a 10" x 15" pan, melt the margarine and stir in the spices, Worcestershire sauce, and lemon juice.

3. Toss in the cereals, crackers, and pretzels to cover evenly.
4. Cook for 45 minutes, stirring occasionally every 15 minutes.
5. Allow to cool on paper towels.
6. Keep in an airtight container.

Tips:

Compare brands—the salt level of cereals, crackers, and pretzels varies widely; always choose the brand with the lowest sodium content.

Nutritional Info; Calories: 92, Protein: 1g, Carbohydrates: 14g, Fat: 3g, Cholesterol: 0mg, Sodium: 127mg, Potassium: 37mg, Phosphorus: 16mg, Calcium: 3 mg, Fiber: 0.4g.

15. A Slew Of Summer Fruits

This wonderful slaw is ideal for persons with diabetes; CKD Stage 1, 2; CKD Stage 3, 4; those on dialysis and CKD 5, and kidney transplant recipients.

Ingredients:

- 1 cleaned apple, stalks, and bottom removed
- 1 washed crisp pear, stalks, and bottom removed

- 1 big stalk cleaned rhubarb, top and bottom removed
- ½ finely sliced red onion
- ½ cup orange juice
- ¼ cup apple cider vinegar
- ½ teaspoons of honey

Preparation:

1. Cut the apples into quarters, avoiding the core and seeds.
2. Then cut those slices into thin, apple matchsticks.
3. Continue with the pears.
4. Finally, cut the rhubarb into quarters, each roughly the same length as your apple and pear matchsticks, and cut those pieces into thin matchsticks as well.

Nutritional   Info;   Calories: 39cal, Carbohydrates: 10g, Dietary Fiber: 1.6g, Protein: 0.4g, Fat: 0.1g, Saturated Fat: 0g, Sodium: 1mg, Potassium: 119mg, Calcium: 14mg, Phosphorus: 12mg.

16. Fruit Salad With Yogurt Dressing

After chilling, persons with diabetes, CKD Stages 1, 2, 3, 4, dialysis, and CKD 5, as well as kidney transplant recipients, can enjoy this delightful and easy-to-make fruit salad.

Ingredients:

- 1 medium apple, skinned
- 10 grapes, green
- 4 ounces drained mandarin oranges in light syrup
- ½ cup pineapple chunks
- ⅓ cup cherry-flavored dried cranberries
- 6 oz. strawberry Greek yogurt
- 6 medium strawberries

Preparation:

1. The apples, grapes, and strawberries should be washed and dried.
2. Cut the apple into bite-size chunks.
3. Strawberries, cut into slices.
4. Combine the apple, grapes, mandarin oranges, pineapple, dried cranberries, and yogurt.
5. Chill for 2 hours, covered.
6. Garnish with cut strawberries and serve.

Nutritional information: Calories 99cal, Carbohydrates 22g, Dietary Fiber 2.4g, Protein 2.6g, Fat 0.7g, Saturated Fat 0.3g, Sodium 12mg, Potassium 161mg, Calcium39 mg, Phosphorus 43mg.

17. Yogurt Feta Vegetable Dip

Ingredients:
- ½ c fat-free Greek yogurt
- ½ c light sour cream
- ¼ c low-fat feta cheese
- 1 tbsp fresh parsley
- 1 tbsp fresh dill
- 2 tsp garlic powder
- 2 tsp onion powder
- 1 tsp ground black pepper

Preparation:
1. Place all items in a food processor or blender and process until smooth.
2. Serve with crunchy veggie sticks like carrots, celery, cucumbers, and bell peppers.

18. Spicy Cornbread

Ingredients:

- 1 cup all-purpose white flour
- 1 cup unbleached cornmeal
- 1 teaspoon sugar
- 2 tsp. baking powder
- 1 tsp. chili powder
- ¼ teaspoon ground black pepper
- 1 cup unenriched rice milk
- 1 egg
- 1 white egg
- 2 tbsp of canola oil
- ½ cup finely chopped scallions
- ¼ cup finely shredded carrots
- 1 minced garlic clove

Preparation:

1. Preheat the oven to 400 degrees Fahrenheit.
2. Stir together flour, cornmeal, sugar, baking powder, chili powder, and pepper in a large mixing bowl.
3. Stir in the rice milk, egg, egg white, and oil until the dry ingredients are barely moistened.
4. Stir scallions, carrots, and garlic into the cornmeal mixture gently.

5. Pour the batter into an 8" square baking pan sprayed with nonstick cooking spray.
6. Bake for 25 to 30 minutes, or until the top begins to turn golden brown, before cutting into eight 2" x 4" pieces.

Tip:

Try onion instead of scallions and red bell pepper instead of carrots for variety.

Nutritional Info; Calories: 188; Protein: 5g; Carbohydrates: 31g; Fat: 5g; Cholesterol: 26mg; Sodium: 155mg; Potassium: 100mg; Phosphorus: 81mg; Calcium: 84mg; Fiber: 2g.

19. Almond Cookies from China

Ingredients:
- 1 cup softened margarine
- 1 cup of sugar
- a single egg
- 3 c. flour
- 1 teaspoon baking soda
- 1 tablespoon almond extract

Preparation:
1. In a medium bowl, blend together cream margarine and sugar.
2. Beat in the egg thoroughly.

3. Sift the dry ingredients into the creamed mixture.
4. Mix in the almond extract thoroughly.
5. Roll the dough into ¾-inch balls.
6. Punch a tiny hole in the middle of each cookie.
7. Bake at 400°F for 10 to 12 minutes, or until the edges of the cookies are golden brown.

Nutritional Info: Calories: 153cal, Carbohydrates: 19.2g, Dietary Fiber: 1.6g, Added Sugar: 8.3g, Protein: 2.2g, Fat: 8g, Saturated Fat: 1.5g, Sodium: 117mg, Potassium: 59mg, Calcium: 6mg, Phosphorus: 57mg.

20. Parfait With Pears And Almonds

This parfait is ideal for people with CKD Stages 1, 2, 3, 4, dialysis, CKD 5, and kidney transplant recipients.

Ingredients:
- 2 quarts rice milk
- ½ cup granulated sugar
- ¼ cup regular flour
- A tsp vanilla extract
- 1 teaspoon almond oil
- 2 peeled and chopped ripe pears

- 4 tablespoons sugar-free strawberry preserves

Preparation:

1. Microwave rice milk for 5 minutes on high in a microwave-safe bowl.
2. Mix the flour and sugar, then add a couple of heaping spoonfuls of the hot rice milk to make a smooth paste.
3. Return the mixture to the heated rice milk and whisk it together.
4. Return the rice milk to the microwave and heat for 1 minute and 30 seconds on high.
5. Cook for 1 minute on high after stirring the mixture with the whip.
6. Remove from the microwave and stir in the almond and vanilla extracts.
7. Place in a shallow dish and chill until cooled.
8. This can be made up to two days in advance.

Nutritional information: 251 calories, 59 grams of carbohydrates, 3.5 grams of dietary fiber, 1.5 grams of protein, 1.4 grams of fat, 0 grams of saturated fat, 49 milligrams of sodium, 170 milligrams of potassium, 154 milligrams of calcium, and 89 milligrams of phosphorus.

21. Mini Wonton Quiche

Ingredients:

- 1 ounce cooked lean ham
- 2 teaspoons chopped green onions
- 2 tbsp red sweet pepper
- 5 medium eggs
- 1 tbsp white all-purpose flour
- 24 wrappers for wontons (3-¼" x 3")

Preparation:

1. Preheat the oven to 350 degrees Fahrenheit.
2. Finely cut the ham, as well as the green onions and red pepper.
3. Set aside. In a medium mixing bowl, combine eggs, ham, onions, pepper, and flour until thoroughly blended.
4. Line 24 mini muffin cups with wonton wrappers, carefully placing the center of 1 wonton wrapper into each cup, allowing ends to overhang above cup corners.
5. Divide the egg mixture evenly among the 24 wonton-lined cups.
6. 12–15 minutes, or until a toothpick inserted near the middle comes out clean.

Tip:

- The little muffin cup is 1-¾" x ¾".
- To minimize cholesterol, use 1-¼ cup low-cholesterol egg product for the eggs.

Nutritional Info; Calories: 70; Protein: 4g; Carbohydrates: 8g; Fat: 2g; Cholesterol: 91mg; Sodium: 95mg; Potassium: 47mg; Phosphorus: 55mg; Calcium: 16mg; Fiber: 0.2g.

22. Crackers With Shrimp Spread

Ingredients:
- ¼ cup softened cream cheese
- 2½ ounces shelled cooked shrimp
- 1 tablespoon ketchup with no additional salt
- a quarter teaspoon Tabasco® spicy sauce
- 1 tsp Worcestershire sauce
- Mrs. Dash® herb seasoning combination, ½ teaspoon
- 24 tiny matzo crackers
- 1 tablespoon fresh parsley

Preparation:
- Allow the cream cheese to soften.
- Combine shrimp and cream cheese in a mixing bowl.

- Combine ketchup, Tabasco sauce, Worcestershire sauce, and Mrs. Dash® herb spice in a mixing bowl.
- Spread 1 teaspoon of spread on each cracker and top with chopped parsley.

Tip:

If preferred, serve with celery sticks instead of crackers.

Nutritional Info; Calories: 57, Protein: 3g, Carbohydrates: 7g, Fat: 1g, Cholesterol: 21mg, Sodium: 69mg, Potassium: 54mg, Phosphorus: 30mg, Calcium: 15mg, Fiber: 0.2g, Added Sugar: 1g.

23. Pretzels Are Addictively Delicious

Ingredients:
- Unsalted pretzels, 32 oz.
- 1-quart canola oil
- 2 tbsp Hidden Valley® Ranch Salad Dressing and Seasoning blend
- a third teaspoon of garlic powder
- 3 tbsp dried dill weed

Preparation:

1. Preheat the oven to 175 degrees Fahrenheit.
2. Spread the pretzels out flat on two 18" x 13" baking sheets, using entire bite-size pretzels or breaking large-size pretzels into pieces.
3. Mix the garlic powder and dill together. Set aside half of the spices. Include the dry salad dressing mix and 3/4 cup canola oil to the other half. Pour evenly over the pretzels and use your hands to make sure the pretzels are thoroughly covered.
4. Bake for 1 hour, rotating the pretzels every 15 minutes.
5. Remove the pretzels from the oven. Let the pretzels cool, then sprinkle with remaining garlic powder, dill weed, and oil. Enjoy!

Tips:

- Snyder's of Hanover brand pretzels were tried in this recipe, but any sort of unsalted pretzel may be used.
- Some kinds of reduced-sodium pretzels include potassium chloride. Check ingredients and avoid them if you are on a low-potassium diet.

- The amount of pretzels in one ounce varies depending on the shape and size. Check the label on the pretzel bag for further information.

Nutritional Info: Calories 176, Protein 3g, Carbohydrates 23g, Fat 8g, Cholesterol 0mg, Sodium 122mg, Potassium 38mg, Phosphorus 44mg, Calcium 13mg, Fiber 0.8g, Added Sugar 0g.

24. Nutty Berry Parfait

Ingredients:
- ½ cup low-fat Greek yogurt
- ¼ cup mixed berries (such as blueberries, strawberries, and raspberries)
- 2 teaspoons chopped walnuts
- 1 teaspoon honey

Preparation:
1. In a glass, place half of the Greek yogurt. Top it with a layer of mixed berries and chopped walnuts.
2. Layers should be repeated.
3. Drizzle honey on top to provide some sweetness.

25. Chickpeas (Roasted)

Ingredients:
- One 15-ounce can of washed and drained chickpeas.
- 1 tablespoon extra virgin olive oil
- 1 teaspoon cumin powder
- ½ tsp smoked paprika
- ¼ tsp garlic powder
- Season with salt to taste

Preparation:
1. Set the oven to 400°F (200°C).
2. To eliminate any excess moisture, use a paper towel to pat the chickpeas dry.
3. Toss chickpeas with olive oil, cumin, smoked paprika, garlic powder, and a touch of salt in a mixing bowl.
4. Spread the chickpeas out in an even layer on a baking sheet.
5. Cook for 20-25 minutes, stirring the pan regularly, until the chickpeas are brown and crispy.
6. Allow to cool before serving as a crispy, protein-packed snack.

26. Protein Bars with a Sweet and Nutty Flavor

Ingredients:

- 2½ cup toasted rolled oats
- ½ cup sliced almonds
- ½ cup ground flaxseed
- ½ oz. peanut butter
- 1 cup dried blueberries, cherries, or Craisins®
- ½ cup of honey

Preparation:

1. To toast the oats, place rolled oats on a baking sheet and bake for 10 minutes, or until golden brown.
2. Mix all of the ingredients until completely combined.
3. Refrigerate for at least one hour or overnight after pressing the protein mixture into a lightly buttered 9" x 9" pan.
4. Serve protein bars cut into appropriate squares.

Nutritional Info; Calories: 283 cal, total fat 13g, saturated fat 2g, trans fat 0g, cholesterol 0mg, sodium 49mg, carbohydrate 39g, protein

7g, phosphorus 177mg, potassium 258mg, dietary fiber 5.8g, calcium 51mg.

27. Lemon Sunburst Bars

Ingredients:
- Crust
- 2 cups regular flour
- ½ cup confectioners' sugar
- 1 cup unsalted butter (2 sticks), room temperature
- Fillings
- 4 eggs
- 1½ cup sugar
- ¼ cup regular flour
- ½ tsp cream of tartar
- ¼ tsp baking soda
- ¼ cup fresh lemon juice

Glaze
- 1 cup sifted powdered sugar
- 2 tbsp of lemon juice

Preparation:
Crust:
1. Preheat the oven to 350 degrees Fahrenheit.
2. Combine the flour, powdered sugar, and 1 cup of softened butter in a large mixing

basin. Mix until the mixture is crumbly. Fill a 9" x 13" baking pan halfway with the ingredients.

3. Bake for a period of 15 to 20 minutes, or until the desired level of browning is achieved.

Filling:

1. In a medium-sized mixing basin, softly whisk the eggs.

2. In a separate dish, whisk together the sugar, flour, cream of tartar, and baking soda. Combine the dry ingredients with the eggs. Whisk in the lemon juice until the egg mixture is slightly thickened.

3. Bake for another 20 minutes, or until the filling is set, over the heated crust.

4. Take the item out of the oven and let it cool.

Glaze:

1. In a small mixing dish, gently combine the lemon juice and powdered sugar until spreadable. As required, adjust the amount of lemon juice.

2. Spread the chilled filling on top. Allow the glaze to set before cutting into 24

bars. Refrigerate any leftover lemon bars.

Nutritional Info: Calories: 200cal, Total Fat 9g, Saturated Fat 5g, Trans Fat 0g, Cholesterol 53mg, Sodium 27mg, Carbohydrates 28g, Protein 2g, Phosphorus 32mg, Potassium 41mg, Dietary Fiber 0.3g, Calcium 9mg.

28. Bites of Carrot Cake

Ingredients:

- 1 pitted date cup
- ½ cup rolled oats, old-fashioned
- ¼ cup pecans, chopped
- ¼ cup of chia seeds
- 2 medium carrots, coarsely chopped (approximately 4 ounces)
- a tsp vanilla extract
- ¾ teaspoon cinnamon powder
- ½ teaspoon ginger powder
- ¼ teaspoon turmeric powder
- ¼ teaspoon of salt
- A pinch of black pepper

Preparation:

1. In a food processor, mix dates, oats, pecans, and chia seeds; pulse until well incorporated and diced.

2. Add carrots, vanilla, cinnamon, ginger, turmeric, salt, and pepper; pulse until well combined and a paste forms.

3. Roll the mixture into 1 tablespoon balls and set aside.

Tips:

Make ahead and store in an airtight jar in the refrigerator for up to 1 week or freeze for up to 3 months.

Nutritional Info: Calories 48cal, Total Fat 1.7g, Saturated Fat 0.2g, Cholesterol 0mg, Sodium 31mg, Total Carbohydrate 8.2g, Protein 0.9g, Phosphorus 34mg, Potassium 87mg, Fiber 1.6g, Calcium 21mg.

29. Citrus Honey Butter Sweet Cornbread Muffins

Ingredients:

- 1 pound cornmeal
- 1 cup of flour
- ½ tablespoon baking soda
- Three tbsp lemon juice
- 1 beaten egg
- 1-quart milk
- ½ pound unsalted butter, melted

- 1 tbsp. vanilla extract
- Honey and butter:
- 2 teaspoons honey
- 1 pound softened unsalted butter
- ½ tsp orange zest
- ¼ tsp black pepper
- ½ tsp orange extract

Preparation:

1. Preheat the oven to 400 degrees Fahrenheit.
2. In a large mixing basin, combine the egg, milk, and butter until thoroughly combined.
3. Separately, combine the flour, cornmeal, and baking soda, then stir into the liquid ingredients until smooth. Make sure not to overestimate.
4. Fill each muffin cup 34 full with muffin liners and bake for 15-20 minutes on the center rack.
5. In a small bowl, mix the honey butter ingredients until smooth; spread on top of cornbread muffins or serve on the side.

Tip:

Make tiny muffins and serve alongside soup or salad.

Nutritional Info: Calories 208, Fat 13g, Saturated Fat 8g, Trans Fat 0g, Cholesterol 48mg, Sodium 179mg, Carbohydrates 20g, Protein 3g, Phosphorus 67mg, Potassium 87mg, Dietary Fiber 1g, Calcium 33mg.

30. Delicious Deviled Eggs

Ingredients:
- 4 big hard-boiled eggs with shells removed
- 2 tbsp mayonnaise (light)
- ½ tsp dried mustard
- ½ teaspoon apple cider vinegar
- 1 tablespoon coarsely chopped onion
- ¼ teaspoon black pepper, ground
- Optional garnish: paprika dash

Preparation:
1. Cut each egg in half lengthwise. Remove the yolks with care and set them in a small dish. On a dish, place the egg white.
2. With a fork, mash the yolks and stir in the mayonnaise, dry mustard, vinegar, onion, and powdered black pepper.

3. Fill cooked egg whites slightly heaping with yolk mixture.
4. Serve the deviled eggs with paprika (optional).
5. Optional: Garnish deviled eggs with paprika before serving.

Nutritional Info: Calories: 98cal, Total Fat 7g, Saturated Fat 2g, Trans Fat 0g, Cholesterol 188mg, Sodium 124mg, Carbohydrates 2g, Protein 6g, Phosphorus 90mg, Potassium 73mg, Dietary Fiber 0g, Calcium 27mg.

31. Coleslaw with Cream

Ingredients:

- 3 tablespoons light mayonnaise
- 3 tbsp. plain nonfat yogurt
- 1 tbsp. Dijon mustard
- 2 tsp apple cider vinegar
- 1 tablespoon sugar
- ½ teaspoon caraway seed (optional) or celery seed
- To taste, season with salt and freshly ground pepper.
- 2 cups shredded red cabbage (about a quarter of a small head)

- 2 cups shredded green cabbage (one-fourth of a small head)
- 2 medium carrots, 1 cup grated

Preparation:

1. In a large mixing bowl, combine the mayonnaise, yogurt, mustard, vinegar, and sugar. If used, sprinkle with caraway (or celery) seed.
2. Season with salt and pepper to taste. Toss in the cabbage and carrots.

Nutritional Info: Calories 48cal, Total Fat 1.5g, Saturated Fat 0.2g, Cholesterol 2mg, Sodium 171mg, Total Carbohydrate 8g, Protein 1.4g, Phosphorus 35mg, Potassium 181mg, Fiber 1.7g, Calcium 44mg.

32. Cakes of Crab

Ingredients:

- Crab meat 120g
- fresh parsley, chopped
- 1 tsp garlic
- ¼ cup red pepper, chopped
- 1 chopped green onion
- 1 egg
- 1 teaspoon lemon juice
- 1 tablespoon bread crumbs

- Black pepper to add flavor
- Oil from vegetables

Preparation:

1. Gently mix together all of the ingredients in a bowl.
2. Make 8 equal portions of the mixture.
3. Form the crab cakes by hand, squeezing off any excess liquid.
4. Heat enough vegetable oil to coat the bottom of a frying pan over medium-high heat.
5. Cook the crab cakes for 2 minutes on each side, or until golden brown.
6. Serve right away.

Nutritional Info: Calories: 75 kcal, Protein: 5g, Carbohydrates: 4g, Fiber: 0.5g, Total Fat: 5g, Sodium: 88mg, Phosphorus: 60mg, Potassium: 116mg.

33. Crostini With Roasted Garlic And Ricotta

Ingredients:

- 6 baguette slices
- 2 tablespoons fresh herbs
- 2 roasted garlic cloves

- black pepper cracked
- 1 pound ricotta cheese

Preparation:

1. Combine the ricotta, herbs, and roasted garlic in a mixing bowl.
2. Spread over baguette slices and broil until crisp.
3. Serve with fresh greens like this Pear and Arugula salad.

Nutritional Info; Calories: 136.5kcal, Protein: 5.8g, Carbohydrates: 20g, Fiber: 1.2g, Total Fat: 3.8g, Sodium: 212mg, Phosphorus: 80mg, Potassium: 97mg.

34. Biscuits Made With Buttermilk

Ingredients:

- 1½ cup all-purpose flour
- 2 teaspoon sugar
- 1 teaspoon baking soda
- 4 tablespoons unsalted butter
- 1 cup of buttermilk

Preparation:

1. Combine the dry ingredients.
2. Cut in the butter until the pieces are the size of peas. To bring the dough together,

add the buttermilk. Spread the dough and shape it into biscuits.

3. Bake at 350°F for 10 minutes, or until brown.

Nutritional Info: Calories: 150 kcal, Protein: 3g, Carbohydrates: 20g, Fibre: 0.6g, Total Fat: 6g, Sodium: 176mg, Phosphorus: 40mg, Potassium: 56mg.

35. Snack Combination

Ingredients:

- 6 tbsp melted margarine
- 2 tbsp. Worcestershire sauce
- ½ teaspoon of seasoning salt
- a quarter teaspoon of garlic powder
- ½ tsp onion powder
- 3 cups of Crispix
- 3 cups of Cheerios
- 3 cup corn feelings
- 1 Kix Cup
- 1 pound pretzels
- 1 cup bagel chips, cut into 1-inch cubes

Preparation:

1. Set the oven to 250 degrees Fahrenheit before beginning to bake.

2. In a large roasting pan, melt margarine. Season to taste. Stir in the remaining ingredients gradually until uniformly covered.

3. 1 hour at a time, stirring every 15 minutes. Allow to cool on paper towels. Keep it in an airtight container.

Nutritional Info; Calories: 88 kcal, Protein: 1.4g, Carbohydrates: 13.7g, Fiber: 0.89g, Total Fat: 3.4g, Sodium: 190mg, Phosphorus: 25.1mg, Potassium: 43.6mg.

36. Delicious Ghanouj

Ingredients:

- 1 big eggplant, halved lengthwise
- 1 garlic head, peeled
- 2 tbsp. (30 mL) olive oil
- To taste, lemon juice

Preparation:

1. Preheat the oven to 350°F with the rack in the middle position. Cover a baking sheet with parchment paper.

2. Place the eggplant on a baking pan, cut side down. Roast until the flesh is extremely soft and easily peels away

from the skin, about 1 hour depending on the size of the eggplant. Allow to cool.

3. Meanwhile, remove the garlic clove tops. Place the cloves in an aluminum foil square. Fold the foil edges up and crimp together to make a firmly sealed packet. Simmer the eggplant for approximately 20 minutes until it is tender. Allow to cool. By pressing the cloves through a garlic press, purée them.

4. Scoop the flesh from the eggplant with a spoon and place it in the bowl of a food processor. Combine the garlic purée, oil, and lemon juice in a mixing bowl. Blend until smooth. Season with pepper to taste.

5. Serve with small pita bread.

Nutritional Info; Calories: 51 kcal, Protein: 1.0g, Carbohydrates: 5.0g, Fiber: 2.4g, Total Fat: 3.6g, Sodium: 2mg, Phosphorus: 22mg, Potassium: 170mg.

37. Tuna Relish

Ingredients:

- 1 can (170 g) drained no-salt-added tuna
- 2 tablespoons light mayonnaise

- 1 teaspoon lemon juice
- 1 teaspoon Dijon mustard
- Season with pepper to taste

Preparation:

1. With a fork, combine all of the ingredients in a mixing dish. Season with pepper to taste. Serve with crackers or bread.

2. To save even more calories, use no-salt-added tuna packaged in water rather than oil.

Nutritional Info: Calories: 101 kcal, Protein: 12.4g, Carbohydrates: 1.3g, Fiber: 0.03g, Total Fat: 4.9g, Sodium: 37mg, Phosphorus: 133 mg, Potassium: 91mg.

38. Bites of Eggplant and Chickpea

Ingredients:

- 3 big eggplants/aubergines, half and scored on the cut side
- Oil for cooking spray
- 2 big peeled garlic cloves
- 2 teaspoon coriander
- 2 teaspoon cumin seeds
- 400g canned chickpeas, washed and drained

- 2 tablespoons chickpea flour
- ½ lemon, both zested and juiced
- 12 lemon slices for serving
- 3 tablespoons polenta

Preparation:

1. Preheat the oven to 200°C/180°C fan/gas 6. Spray the eggplant halves well with oil before placing them cut-side up in a large roasting pan with the garlic, coriander, and cumin seeds. Season with salt and pepper, then roast for 40 minutes, or until the eggplant is soft. Allow to cool slightly.

2. Remove the peels off the eggplant and scoop the meat into a basin. Scrape the spices and garlic into the bowl with a spatula. Mash together the chickpeas, chickpea flour, lemon zest, and juice, and season to taste. Don't worry if the mixture is a little mushy; it will firm up in the refrigerator.

3. Form the mixture into 20 balls and place them on a baking sheet lined with parchment paper. Refrigerate for at least 30 minutes.

4. Preheat the oven to 180°C/160°C fan/gas 4. Place the polenta on a dish, roll the

balls in it to coat, then return to the tray and lightly oil each one. Cook for 20 minutes, or until crisp, hot, and golden. With lemon slices on the side, serve.

Tip:

The recipe goes great with the harissa yogurt dip.

Nutritional Info: Calories: 72 kcal, Protein: 3g, Carbohydrates: 18g, Fibre: 4g, Total Fat: 1g, Sodium: 63 mg, Phosphorus: 36mg, Potassium: 162mg.

39. *Beef Jerky*

Ingredients:

- 3 lbs. moose rump meat
- ¼ cup low-sodium soy sauce
- ½ teaspoon garlic powder
- ½ teaspoon onion powder
- ½ teaspoon pepper
- 2 tablespoons hickory liquid smoke

Preparation:

1. Trim fat from the edges of the Moose roast and slice it into 12-inch thick pieces.
2. Combine reduced-sodium soy sauce, garlic powder, onion powder, pepper, and

hickory liquid smoke in a large mixing bowl and toss until all of the meat is covered in the marinade.

3. Allow the mixture to chill in the refrigerator for a minimum of 6 hours, ideally overnight.
4. Preheat the oven to 200°F.
5. Wrap 1 big pan with foil and distribute moose strips on it. Cook for 2 hours.
6. After baking, remove the jerky from the oven and allow it to cool fully.

Nutritional Info: Calories: 68 kcal, Protein: 14 g, Carbohydrates: 0.7 g, Total Fat: 0.9 g, Sodium: 201.2mg, Phosphorus: 102.61mg, Potassium: 198.16mg.

40. Dinner Rolls (hamburger buns) with Low Sodium

Ingredients:
- 1 cup + 2 tbsp heated (110F to 115F) water
- a third of a cup of oil
- 2 tablespoons active dry yeast
- 2 tablespoons sugar
- 1 big egg

- 3½ cups all-purpose flour (bread flour can also be used)

Preparation:

1. Preheat the oven to 400°F.
2. Combine the water, oil, yeast, and sugar in a medium mixing basin. Allow to stand for 15 minutes, or until extremely frothy.
3. Gently fold in the egg and 2 cups of the flour.
4. Stir in the remaining flour, ½ cup at a time, until all of it is mixed and a dough forms.
5. On a sheet pan, shape the dough into 12 equal rolls (flatten slightly for hamburger buns). Allow rolls to rest for 10 minutes.
6. Bake for 10-15 minutes in a preheated oven or until golden brown.

Nutritional Info; Calories: 206.7kcal, Protein: 5.1g, Carbohydrates: 30.8g, Fiber: 1.6g, Total Fat: 6.9g, Sodium: 7.8mg, Phosphorus: 59.28mg, Potassium: 63.4mg.

41. Pizza with Roasted Red Bell Peppers and Cauliflower

Ingredients:

- ½ cauliflower head, stalk removed
- ¼ cup grated parmesan cheese
- 1 teaspoon turmeric
- 1 tablespoon of Italian seasoning
- ¼ teaspoon salt
- 1 egg
- ½ cup mozzarella cheese, shredded
- 2 ripe red bell peppers
- 1 tablespoon olive oil plus 1 tablespoon for pouring on peppers and garlic
- 2-3 garlic cloves, peeled
- 5 fresh basil sprigs
- 1 teaspoon corn (or potato) starch

Preparation:

1. Preheat the oven to 450 degrees Fahrenheit.
2. Wash and pat dry the bell peppers, then place them on a baking sheet with the unpeeled garlic cloves (this prevents the garlic from burning).

3. Drizzle with 1 tsp oil, season with salt and bake for 30 minutes, or until the red bell peppers are soft and brown.
4. While the peppers are baking, pulse the cauliflower in a food processor until it is crumbly and has a rice-like texture.
5. Line a baking sheet with parchment paper, then spread the riced cauliflower in a single layer and bake for 15 minutes under the bell peppers and garlic in the same oven.
6. Keep an eye on the red bell peppers and garlic. When it's done, remove it from the oven and set it aside for 10 minutes to cool.
7. Peel the peppers and garlic, and remove the stems.
8. In a food processor, blend the peppers, garlic, olive oil, and cornstarch until finely pureed and smooth.
9. Set aside the bell pepper sauce after stirring it for 10-15 minutes on low heat until it thickens.
10. Remove the cauliflower from the oven and, once cold, transfer the riced cauliflower to a clean cheesecloth or dish towel.

11. Squeeze off any extra moisture and discard it.
12. Combine the riced cauliflower, spices, parmesan, salt, and egg in a large mixing basin. Combine thoroughly.
13. Form the dough into a ¼-inch-thick circle and place it on a baking sheet coated with parchment paper.
14. Bake at 400^0F for 30 minutes, or until brown. Bake for 10 minutes more after flipping the crust.
15. Remove from the oven and top with the roasted red pepper sauce, mozzarella, and basil.
16. Bake for another 5-10 minutes, or until the cheese melts.
17. This recipe yields two little pizzas! Slice and serve!

Nutritional Info; Calories: 325Kcal, Protein: 20g, Carbohydrates: 9g, Fiber: 2g, Total Fat: 22g, Sodium: 382mg, Phosphorus: 372mg, Potassium: 438mg.

42. Vegan Kid-Friendly Kimchi

Ingredients:

- 1 napa cabbage head (1 pound)

- 4 green onion stems, chopped into bits (green portion only)
- 3 tablespoons red pepper flakes
- ½ cup finely sliced onions
- 4 cloves of garlic, minced
- 1 inch of ginger, grated
- 1 tsp sugar
- 2 tablespoons sea salt

Preparation:

1. Cut the cabbage into 8 wedges vertically. In a sizable bowl, mix together the wedges. Massage 2 tbsp salt into the cabbage until moist and slightly wilted, 3-4 minutes. Set the timer for 50 minutes.

2. In the meantime, prepare the remaining ingredients. Slice ½ cup onions thinly. Green onion greens should be cut into 2-inch chunks. 4 garlic cloves, minced. 1 inch fresh ginger, grated. Combine minced garlic and grated ginger with 1 teaspoon sugar to make a paste.

3. After 50 minutes, place the cabbage in a colander and thoroughly rinse it under cold running water for 1 minute. Allow cabbage to drain for 30 minutes.

4. Combine cabbage, sliced onions, green onion pieces, garlic ginger paste, and 3 tablespoons red pepper flakes in a large mixing dish. Mix until all of the ingredients are properly blended.

5. Fill clean jars halfway with the mixture, leaving 1 inch at the top for fermentation. Place on the counter for 3 days at room temperature before transferring to the fridge for up to many months of storage. Fermentation will continue in the refrigerator.

6. After 3 days, the top of the kimchi may seem frothy or contain little bubbles, indicating fermentation. If the kimchi stinks or appears slimy, the fermentation was most likely unsuccessful; trash and restart.

Nutritional Information: 2Kcal, 111mg sodium, 2mg phosphorus, and 9mg potassium.

43. Dip with Curried Eggplant

Ingredients:
- 1 medium roasted eggplant
- 1 tablespoon lemon juice
- 2 garlic cloves

- 2 teaspoons curry powder
- ¼ teaspoon ginger
- ¼ cup cilantro, fresh

Preparation:

1. Cut the eggplants in half and score them.
2. Drizzle with olive oil and roast at 350°F for 45-60 minutes, or until the flesh is tender.
3. Remove the meat and discard the skins.
4. In a food processor, combine all ingredients until smooth.
5. Serve alongside baked pita chips.

Nutritional Info; Calories: 23Kcal, Protein: 1g, Carbohydrates: 5g, Fiber: 3g, Sodium: 2.4mg, Phosphorus: 23.5mg, Potassium: 198mg.

44. Herbed Biscuits from Scratch

Looking for some kidney-friendly biscuits? We have the recipe. All you need are herbs, flour, and milk to make these moist and delicious biscuits that are full of fresh-from-the-oven pleasure.

Ingredients:

- 1¼ cup all-purpose flour
- 1 teaspoon tartar sauce
- ½ tsp baking soda

- 1/4 cup of mayonnaise
- 13% skim milk
- 3 tablespoons chives or any herb of choice, fresh or dried
- Nonstick cooking spray

Preparation:

1. Preheat the oven to 400 degrees Fahrenheit. Spray a cookie sheet with nonstick cooking spray next.
2. In a large mixing basin, combine the flour, cream of tartar, and baking soda. Then, using a fork, stir in the mayonnaise until the mixture resembles coarse cornmeal.
3. Combine the milk and herbs in a separate bowl, then add to the flour mixture. Stir until everything is mixed.
4. Place a heaping spoonful of the mixture on the cookie sheet. 10 minutes in the oven.
5. Store in the fridge until you are ready to use it.

Nutritional Info; Calories: 109cal, Total Fat 4g, Saturated Fat 1g, Trans Fat 0g, Cholesterol 2mg, Sodium 88mg, Carbohydrates 15g, Protein 3g, Phosphorus 34 mg, Potassium 85 mg, Dietary Fiber 1g, Calcium 21mg.

45. Crab Dip with Hot Sauce

Ingredients:

- Softened cream cheese, 18 oz (250 mL)
- 1 tablespoon finely minced onion
- 1 teaspoon lemon juice
- 2 tablespoons Worcestershire sauce
- ⅛ teaspoon black pepper
- To taste, cayenne pepper
- 2 tablespoons milk or unsweetened rice beverage
- 16 oz rinsed can of crab meat

Preparation:

1. Set the oven to 375°F (190°C).
2. In a mixing bowl, combine the cream cheese. Add the onion, lemon juice, Worcestershire sauce, black and cayenne peppers, and salt and pepper to taste. Combine thoroughly. Mix in the milk/rice beverage. Stir in the crab meat until well combined.
3. Put the mixture in an oven-safe dish. Cook for 15 minutes, or until the dish is heated through and bubbling. Serve heated with pita bread triangles or low-sodium crackers.

OR

4. Microwave for 4 minutes, stirring every 1-2 minutes, until the mixture is heated and bubbling.

Nutritional Info: Calories: 98Kcal, Protein: 5g, Carbohydrates: 2g, Fiber: 2g, Total Fat: 8g, Sodium: 132mg, Phosphorus: 61mg, Potassium: 91mg.

46. Bites of Cucumber Cream Cheese

Ingredients:
- 1 medium cucumber, thinly sliced
- 2 tbsp cream cheese (low sodium)
- Dill, fresh, chopped (for garnish)
- Season with salt and pepper to taste.

Preparation:
1. On each cucumber round, spread a thin layer of low-sodium cream cheese.
2. Season the cream cheese with salt and pepper to taste.
3. Garnish with fresh dill, if desired.
4. These creamy cucumber nibbles are a light, kidney-friendly snack.

47. Cucumber Salad, Cool and Crispy

Cool, crunchy, and simple. Chill sliced cucumbers with sodium-free Italian dressing and freshly ground black pepper before serving.

Ingredients:

- 2 cups fresh cucumber (sliced into 14-inch pieces, optional peeling)
- 2 tablespoons salad dressing (Italian or Caesar)
- To taste, freshly ground black pepper

Preparation:

1. Combine cucumber and salad dressing in a medium-sized bowl with a cover.
2. Cover with the lid and shake to coat.
3. Season with freshly ground black pepper. Refrigerate.
4. It is best served chilled.

<u>Nutritional Info;</u> Calories: 27cal, Total Fat: 2g, Cholesterol: 0mg, Sodium: 74mg, Carbohydrates: 3g, Protein: 0g, Phosphorus: 14mg, Potassium: 90mg, Dietary Fiber: 0g, Calcium: 12mg.

47. Salad with Crunchy Quinoa

The nutty flavor of protein-packed quinoa is combined with tomatoes, cucumbers, green onions, fresh mint, and parsley in this crisp, colorful quinoa salad. Pour the salad into Bibb lettuce leaf "cups" for an extra cool crunch.

Ingredients:

- 1 cup washed quinoa
- 2 c. water
- 5 diced cherry tomatoes
- ½ cup seeded and sliced cucumbers
- 3 chopped green onions
- ¼ cup chopped fresh mint
- ½ cup chopped flat-leaf parsley
- 2 tbsp. fresh lemon juice
- 1 tablespoon lemon zest (grated)
- four tbsp olive oil
- ¼ cup grated parmesan cheese
- ½ head of Boston or Bibb lettuce, divided into cups

Preparation:

1. Rinse the quinoa under cold running water until it is clear, then drain well.
2. Toast the quinoa in a skillet over medium-high heat for 2 minutes, turning constantly. Bring to a boil with 2 cups of

water. Reduce the heat to low, cover the pan, and leave to cook for 8-10 minutes. Allow to cook before fluffing with a fork.

3. Combine the herbs, lemon juice, zest, and olive oil with the tomatoes, cucumbers, and onions. To the mixture, add the chilled quinoa.

4. Spoon the mixture into lettuce cups and top with parmesan cheese.

Nutritional Info; Calories: 158cal, Total Fat: 9g, Cholesterol: 2mg, Sodium: 46mg, Carbohydrates: 16g, Protein: 5g, Phosphorus: 129mg, Potassium: 237mg, Dietary Fiber: 2.3g, Calcium: 61mg.

48. Dip with Smoky and Savory Salmon

This smoked salmon dip recipe is rich and savory, and it makes an excellent appetizer or side dish.

Ingredients:

- 1 pound fresh skinless and boneless fish, sliced into four pieces
- 2 tsp. smoked paprika

- 1 cup softened cream cheese
- ¼ cups capers
- ¼ cup lemon juice and half a lemon zest (approximately 1 teaspoon)
- 2 teaspoons finely diced red onions
- 1 teaspoon black pepper, ground
- 1 tablespoon chopped fresh parsley

Preparation:

1. Poach the fish for 4-6 minutes over medium-high heat in 2 cups of water and 1 teaspoon of smoked paprika; the pot should be covered but not come to a boil. Remove from the oven and cool for at least 30 minutes.

2. Mix in the remaining ingredients until smooth. Fold the salmon into the cream cheese mixture in bite-sized chunks.

3. Refrigerate the salmon dip for 20-30 minutes. Serve with celery sticks, corn chips, and carrots, or wrap in an iceberg lettuce leaf.

Nutritional Info: Calories: 133cal, Total Fat 9g, Saturated Fat 4g, Trans Fat 0g, Cholesterol 43mg, Sodium 147mg, Carbohydrates 2g, Protein 10g, Phosphorus 110 mg, Potassium 259 mg, Dietary Fiber 0mg, Calcium 28mg.

49. Dill Yogurt Zucchini Fritters

Ingredients:

- ½ pound grated zucchini
- 1⅛ tsp kosher salt, divided
- ⅓ cup plain whole-milk Greek yogurt
- 2 tbsp. soured cream
- 2 tbsp fresh dill, chopped
- 1 tbsp. sherry vinegar
- 1 teaspoon water
- ½ teaspoon freshly grated lemon zest
- a quarter teaspoon of ground pepper, divided
- 1 big beaten egg
- ⅓ cup regular flour
- 1¼ cup cornmeal
- 2 tbsp extra virgin olive oil

Preparation:

1. Toss the zucchini in a fine-mesh sieve with ⅛ teaspoon salt. Allow for a 15-minute resting period.

2. Meanwhile, in a small mixing bowl, combine the yogurt, sour cream, dill, vinegar, water, lemon zest, and ¼ teaspoon salt and pepper. Place aside.

3. Squeeze the zucchini in a clean dish towel until dry. In a large mixing basin,

combine the egg, flour, cornmeal, ½ teaspoon salt, and the remaining ½ teaspoon pepper.

4. In a sizable nonstick pan over medium-high heat, warm 1 tablespoon of oil. Drop 6 fritters onto the pan and flatten with a spatula into 2-inch disks, using 2 teaspoons of the zucchini mixture for each. Cook until golden brown on both sides, about 2 minutes on each side. Place on a wire rack to cool. Rep with the rest of the zucchini mixture and 1 tablespoon oil. Sprinkle the remaining ¼ teaspoon salt over the fritters. Serve right away with the saved sauce.

Nutritional Info: Calories 105, Total Fat 5.7g, Saturated Fat 1.4g, Cholesterol 26mg, Sodium 292mg, Carbohydrate 10.3g, Protein 3.7g, Phosphorus 77mg, Potassium 270mg, Fiber 1.2g, Calcium 33mg.

50. Smoothie with Chocolate

In virtually no time, you can make a fast liquid supper. Combine condensed and evaporated milk, cinnamon, nutmeg, ice, and chocolate-flavored whey protein in a blender.

Ingredients:

- 2 scoops whey protein with chocolate flavor
- 2 cups of ice
- ½ cup drained evaporated milk
- ¼ cup sweetened condensed milk
- ¼ teaspoon cinnamon powder
- 1 tsp. nutmeg

Preparation:

1. In a blender, combine all ingredients except the cinnamon and process on high for 1-2 minutes, or until smooth.
2. To serve, top with whipped cream and sprinkle with cinnamon.

Nutritional Info; Calories: 142cal, Total Fat: 4g, Saturated Fat: 3g, Trans Fat: 0g, Cholesterol: 18mg, Sodium: 134mg, Carbohydrates: 17g, Protein: 10g, Phosphorus: 162mg, Potassium: 247mg, Dietary Fiber: 0.9g, Calcium: 204mg.

51. Dip with Spicy Black Beans

Ingredients:

- One-half of a cup of can black beans, without any added salt.
- ¼ cup fat-free Greek yogurt
- 1 ounce lime juice (from 1 lime)
- ½ teaspoon cumin
- ½ teaspoon oregano
- ½ teaspoon garlic powder
- ¼ teaspoon cayenne pepper
- 2 tablespoons olive oil
- ¼ cup fresh cilantro
- ¼ cup finely chopped onion

Preparation:

- Mix all the ingredients in a food processor or blender until a homogeneous consistency is achieved.
- Top with some salsa, fat-free yogurt, and fresh cilantro.
- Cold or hot, serve with chips or veggie sticks...or in a taco!

"A healthy snack is a small investment with big returns – a vibrant life filled with wellness and joy."

CHAPTER 4

Nutrient Balance Planning

Planning for nutritional balance is the compass directing you towards a gastronomic adventure that feeds both body and spirit in the complicated dance of renal diet snacking. It's not only about making tasty snacks; it's about making sure each mouthful contributes to a balanced nutritional profile.

1. Protein Expertise

Proteins are key building blocks, and including them in your snacks ensures that you have prolonged energy and satiety. Choose lean proteins like chicken or fish, or plant-based options like beans and lentils. This not only meets your body's amino acid requirements, but it also coincides with the renal diet's emphasis on limiting phosphorus consumption.

2. Fiber Consumption

Fiber, the hidden hero, is essential in renal diet snacks. Incorporate fiber-rich whole grains, fruits, and vegetables to improve digestive health and a constant flow of energy. This balance promotes satiety, prevents overeating, and ensures that your snacks are both kidney-friendly and enjoyable.

3. Navigating the Lipid Landscape with Heart-Healthy Fats

While fats should be consumed in moderation, choosing heart-healthy choices such as avocados, olive oil, and almonds adds a rich and fulfilling touch to your snacking. These fats not only add to a well-rounded taste profile, but they also support cardiovascular health, which is important for individuals dealing with renal disease.

4. Hydration Balance

Hydration is the subtle thread that knits everything together in the fabric of nutritional balance. To contribute to your regular fluid intake without overburdening your kidneys, choose snacks with high water content, such as fresh fruits and vegetables. This provides not just flavor but also a modest yet important contribution to your general health.

Tips for Portion Control

Portion control is the unseen architect who ensures your snacks match your taste preferences as well as your kidney health goals.

It's about enjoying the moment without going overboard, establishing a fine balance that elevates nibbles to a conscious culinary experience.

1. Divide and Conquer

Pre-portioning before dipping into your snack hoard is a simple yet efficient method. Snacks should be divided into single-serving portions. This not only helps with portion management, but it also avoids the temptation of continual snacking, ensuring that each meal corresponds with your nutritional goals.

2. Mindful Eating

Eating is a sensory experience, not a sprint. Mindful eating is enjoying each meal and appreciating the flavors and sensations. This method allows your brain to detect satisfaction, lowering the probability of overeating and encouraging a conscious relationship with your food.

3. Balanced Bites

Changing up your snack options offers a balanced food intake and reduces boredom. Instead of reaching for the same snack over and over, broaden your options. This not only caters to your taste preferences, but it also broadens your nutritional intake, improving your overall health.

4. Strategic Snacking Requires Timing

Strategic snacking is matching your snack consumption to your daily activity and schedule. Plan snacks around moments of increased energy expenditure or when hunger strikes, making sure that each food serves a function in fuelling your body and minimizing excessive hunger.

5. Beverage Awareness

Beverages are sometimes ignored when it comes to portion control. Be aware of liquid calories and choose hydrating options such as water or herbal teas. This not only increases your overall fluid intake but also keeps you from consuming too many calories from sugary beverages.

Identifying and Replacing High-Sodium Offenders

Navigating the panorama of high-sodium culprits in the area of renal diet snacks becomes a critical skill for persons interested in prioritizing kidney health. The ability to detect these hidden salt sources and effortlessly swap them in snack recipes offers a pleasant journey without jeopardizing renal health.

1. Snacks that have been processed and packaged:

In processed and packaged treats, the attraction of convenience frequently conceals a sodium-heavy reality. Chips, crackers, and even seemingly harmless pretzels can contain high levels of salt. Reading food labels for salt levels and choosing low-sodium alternatives become necessary behaviors.

2. Soups And Broths In Cans:

While a hot bowl of soup is soothing, canned soups sometimes disguise high salt levels. Individuals may enjoy the heartiness of soup without the salt excess by locating low-sodium broth or, better yet, producing homemade broth.

3. Deli Meats with Cheese:

Cheese and deli meats, both popular snack foods, can be rich in salt. Lower-sodium cheeses and fresh, lean protein sources such as grilled chicken or turkey give tasty alternatives.

4. Sauces And Condiments:

Sauces and condiments are infamous for sneaking additional salt into the diet. Soy sauce, ketchup, and salad dressings are common causes. Individuals can keep the flavor without losing renal health by investigating low-sodium choices or creating homemade alternatives.

5. Bakery Products:

Baked foods, such as bread and pastries, may have higher salt levels than expected. Those who enjoy baked snacks must choose low-sodium bread or experiment with homemade alternatives prepared with renal-friendly components.

Creating Kidney-Friendly Flavor by Substituting High-Sodium Culprits

1. Snacks Made at Home:

Taking control of your salt consumption is the most effective method. Making homemade snacks allows people to carefully pick each item, including low-sodium options and herbs for taste improvement.

2. Selecting Fresh Produce:

Including fresh fruits and vegetables in snacks not only increases nutritional value but also has a low salt content. Fresh produce adds natural sweetness and crunch to snacks, making them a delicious and kidney-friendly alternative to processed alternatives.

3. Spices And Herbs:

For renal diet fans, the world of herbs and spices is a treasure trove. Experimenting with fragrant herbs like basil, rosemary, and thyme, as well as spices like cumin and paprika, allows people to flavor food without relying on salt.

4. Smart Ingredient Substitutions:

Smart ingredient adjustments may make a big impact. Choosing low-sodium broths, substituting potassium-rich alternatives such as applesauce in baking, and choosing homemade dressings over store-bought ones are all smart plays in the search for kidney-friendly eating.

5. Conscious Condiment Selections:

Rather than avoiding condiments entirely, making informed selections is essential. Choosing low-sodium soy sauce, experimenting with vinegar-based dressings, and making homemade salsa all present chances for savory condiments that support renal health.

Managing Potassium and Phosphorus Intake

Managing intake becomes a critical skill in the delicate dance of renal diet snacking, especially when navigating the potential hazards of potassium and phosphorus. The precise balance of these minerals is critical for those with kidney problems, and knowing how to prevent excess consumption of snack foods is an important part of preserving renal health.

Potassium Pitfalls:

1. Bananas and oranges should be avoided:

While fruits are a healthy snack option, high-potassium fruits such as bananas and oranges can tip the scales. Lower-potassium fruits such as berries, apples, or grapes can be used in snack dishes for a sweet twist without the potassium overdose.

2. Limit Your Intake Of Nuts And Seeds:

While nuts and seeds are high in nutrients, they can also lead to high potassium levels. Managing consumption entails eating smaller quantities or looking for alternatives in snack dishes, such as sunflower seeds, which have a lower potassium concentration.

3. Dairy Use with Caution:

Dairy products are high in potassium, and too much of it can be harmful. When creating snack dishes, consider using low-potassium dairy products or non-dairy alternatives such as almond or rice milk.

4. Be Wary of Potassium Additives:

Potassium additions in processed and packaged foods may contribute to concealed potassium consumption. Managing this entails carefully reading labels and selecting foods with little or no potassium additions.

The Phosphorus Pitfalls:

1. Caution is advised: Dairy and Protein:

Phosphorus is commonly found in dairy and protein-rich meals. Managing consumption necessitates taking precautions, such as selecting low-phosphorus dairy choices and lean protein sources when adding them to snack meals.

2. Whole Grains in Moderation:

While whole grains are nutritious, they can be rich in phosphorus. Managing consumption entails limiting the use of whole grains in snack recipes or, in certain situations, investigating lower-phosphorus substitutes such as white rice or refined flour.

3. Keep an eye out for colas and dark sodas:

Colas and dark sodas can have significant levels of phosphorus additions, making them a hidden source of phosphorus. To satiate thirst without jeopardizing kidney health, choose phosphorus-free or low-phosphorus beverage options in snack recipes.

4. Limit your intake of processed foods:

For preservation, phosphorus additions are frequently included in processed and convenience foods. To control consumption, make a conscious effort to avoid using highly processed foods in snack dishes, instead opting for fresh and whole products.

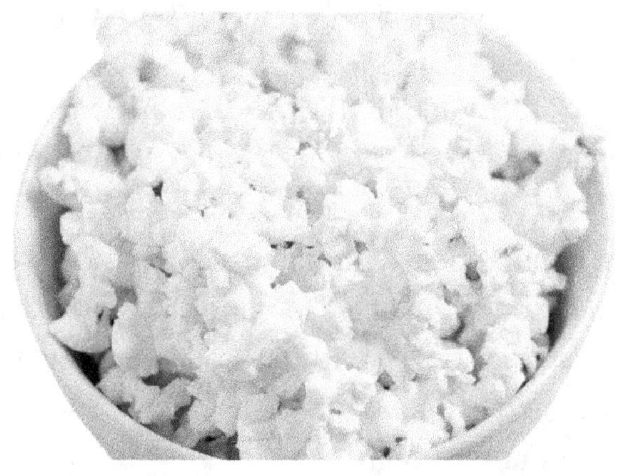

CHAPTER 5

Intake Management Techniques in Snack Recipes

1. Portion Management:

Portion control is an all-purpose method for controlling potassium and phosphorus consumption in snack foods. Individuals can enjoy a variety of snacks without exceeding acceptable mineral levels by controlling serving quantities.

2. Snack Options Should Be Diversified:

Diversifying snack options, rather than relying mainly on a single food, helps to disperse potassium and phosphorus consumption. This method allows people to enjoy a variety of tastes and nutrients without concentrating too many minerals in one food.

3. Homemade Delights:

Individuals who choose homemade snacks have more control over the components and their amounts. This method allows for deliberate choices concerning potassium and phosphorus sources, ensuring that snacks fit with kidney health goals.

4. Speak with a Dietitian:

When in doubt, consulting a renal dietician is helpful. These experts may give tailored advice, assisting individuals in managing their unique dietary requirements and navigating the difficulties of potassium and phosphorus in snack meals.

Frequently Asked Questions

Individuals frequently meet nutritional questions and culinary issues in the complex terrain of renal diet snacks, which need careful analysis and creative solutions. This subchapter tries to address frequent renal diet problems by giving ideas on creating kidney-friendly snacks without sacrificing flavor or nutritional value.

1. *How Can I Make Snack Recipes More Nutritious?*

Balanced nutrition in renal diet snacks requires careful ingredient selection. To guarantee a wide range of nutrients, include a mix of fruits, vegetables, lean meats, and whole grains. A fruit and nut parfait or vegetable sticks with hummus, for example, provide a good source of vitamins, minerals, and fiber.

2. What Are Good Protein Options for Kid-Friendly Snacks?

It is critical to choose lean protein sources. Excellent options include grilled chicken, turkey, hard-boiled egg whites, and hummus. These proteins not only help with snack satiety, but they also support kidney health objectives.

3. How Can I Increase Fiber Intake in Snacks Without Increasing Phosphorus Intake?

Selecting low-phosphorus fiber sources can help to balance fiber consumption while regulating phosphorus. Include veggies such as bell peppers, cucumbers, and zucchini, and select healthy grains with care. Fiber-rich and phosphorus-conscious snack alternatives include whole-grain crackers with guacamole or quinoa salad.

4. Are Kidney-Friendly Sweeteners Available for Baking Snacks?

There are kidney-friendly sweeteners available. To sweeten snacks without relying on typical sugars, use alternatives such as stevia or monk fruit. In addition, using naturally sweet fruits like berries or apples in baking recipes adds a sweet twist without adding too much sugar.

5. How Can I Make Sure I'm Getting Enough Fluids Through Snacks?

Fluid-friendly foods aid with hydration. Include water-rich snacks, such as watermelon skewers or cucumber salad. Herbal teas or infused water may also be delicious beverage options to accompany food and aid with hydration.

6. How Can I Fit Renal Diet Snacks Into My Busy Schedule?

Incorporating renal diet snacks into a hectic lifestyle necessitates forethought and deliberate selections. Prepare quick-grab items such as pre-cut fruits, low-sodium trail mix, or portioned yogurt cups. Choose products that are easy to transport, such as unsalted crackers with hummus or sliced veggies with a small jar of dip.

Keep kidney-friendly snacks on hand at work, in your bag, or your car. Cook snacks in bulk, such as boiled eggs, and keep them in the fridge for easy consumption.

Choose snacks that are easy to transport, such as unsalted almonds, low-sodium cheese sticks, or homemade protein bars. You may maintain a renal-friendly diet even if your schedule is hectic if you plan your snacks ahead of time.

7. *Is it possible to get pre-packaged snacks that are suitable for a renal diet?*

Yes, there are pre-packaged snacks that are renal-friendly. Look for low salt, phosphorus, and potassium alternatives. Unsalted rice cakes, low-sodium popcorn, portion-controlled nut packs, and low-potassium fruit cups (in moderation) are all safe bets.

Sodium, potassium, and phosphorus levels should always be checked on nutrition labels. Keep in mind that while homemade snacks give you greater control over the contents, diligent label reading can help you identify practical pre-packaged choices that meet your renal dietary needs. It is best to get tailored advice from a healthcare practitioner or a dietician.

8. *How Do I Adjust My Renal Diet Snack Intake If I Exercise Regularly?*

If you include frequent activity in your routine while on a renal diet, you may need to adapt your snack consumption accordingly. Exercise can raise your energy expenditure and dietary requirements. Consume renal-friendly snacks with a combination of carbs and protein to help with energy levels and muscle repair.

Consider having a short snack before exercise to provide a rapid supply of energy, followed by a protein-rich snack to help in recuperation. Keep an eye on your hydration and electrolyte balance. A nutritionist who is acquainted with renal nutrition can assist you in tailoring your snack plan to your workout regimen and specific needs.

9. Can I Have a Cheat Day on a Renal Diet, and How Does It Affect My Snack Selections?

While occasional treats can be included in a renal diet, they must be used with caution. A cheat day might throw off your careful dietary balance and jeopardize your kidney health. If you must indulge, consider low-potassium, low-phosphorus goodies and account for them in your overall nutritional consumption.

Balance is crucial, and choosing renal-friendly snacks even on cheat days will help you stick to your nutritional objectives. Consultation with a nutritionist will ensure that your selections are in line with your health demands, minimizing the strain on your kidneys but allowing for occasional indulgences.

10. What Are Some Kidney-Friendly Snacks That Also Meet Other Dietary Restrictions, Such as Gluten-Free or Vegan?

Several kidney-friendly foods are gluten-free and vegan-friendly. Fresh fruits, veggie sticks with hummus, rice cakes with almond butter, gluten-free crackers with dairy-free cheese, mixed nuts, chia seed pudding prepared with almond milk, and quinoa salad with vegetables are among the available options.

By concentrating on full, unadulterated foods, these options appeal to renal, gluten-free, and vegan needs. Always check labels and talk with a nutritionist to ensure that your snacks suit your individual nutritional needs while also promoting kidney health and general well-being.

Success Strategies

1. Plan Ahead Of Time:

Planning is essential for success. Plan snack menus ahead of time to anticipate nutritional needs and potential cooking challenges. This not only speeds up the cooking process but also ensures that nutritional objectives are met.

2. Experiment And Invent:

Renal diet snacks provide a blank canvas for culinary exploration. Be willing to experiment with new ingredients, flavors, and cooking techniques. Experimenting keeps snacks interesting while also expanding the repertoire of kidney-friendly recipes.

3. Seek Professional Help:

A consultation with a renal dietician gives tailored advice. A dietitian may provide insight into individual dietary needs, address concerns, and make specific recommendations for creating snacks that support renal health objectives.

4. Accept Community and Resources:

Joining renal diet networks or gaining access to credible resources may give a wealth of information and support. Individuals on their renal diet journey might benefit from learning from the experiences of others, exchanging recipes, and finding reputable information.

5. Culinary Achievements Should Be Celebrated:

Every renal diet snack that is effectively created is a culinary achievement. Celebrate these accomplishments, no matter how minor.

Recognizing and appreciating the effort put forth in preparing kidney-friendly snacks promotes a good attitude and encourages commitment to renal health.

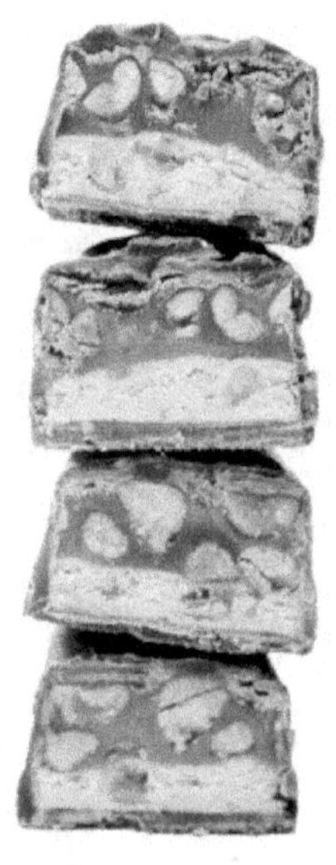

"Nourishing your body with kidney-friendly snacks is not just a choice; it's a celebration of your health and resilience."

CONCLUSION

As you Conclude this book, Remember that having a happy outlook is just as important as picking kidney-friendly items as you finish this renal diet-snacking journey.

Celebrating tiny triumphs, appreciating the learning curve, and relishing the delight of creating great snacks that prioritize your health are all ways to stay happy on the renal diet path. Whether you're experimenting with new flavors or adjusting old favorites, each step demonstrates your dedication to kidney health. Allow positivity to lead you as you continue to discover the wide and delightful world of renal diet snacks.

Your commitment to a kidney-friendly lifestyle is a celebration of perseverance, inventiveness, and the pursuit of a delectable and health-conscious culinary experience.

Dear Reader,

Thank you for embarking on the Renal Diet Snacks adventure with me. Your dedication to kidney health is truly inspiring. I hope this culinary journey brings both joy and nourishment to your life. Your commitment to exploring kidney-friendly snacks is commendable, and I'm grateful for the opportunity to be a part of your health-conscious culinary exploration.

With heartfelt appreciation,

Nancy K. Doctor

BONUS: 2-WEEKS SNACK MEAL PLAN

<u>Week 1:</u>

Day 1:

- Breakfast: Ginger Soft Cookies
- Lunch: Baked Pita Crisps with Tuna Relish
- Dinner: Soup with Sour Cherries from Hungary

Day 2:

- Breakfast: Bars of Granola
- Lunch: Sweet & Sour Meatballs
- Dinner: Chickpeas (Roasted) with Herbed Biscuits

Day 3:

- Breakfast: Fruit Crisp
- Lunch: Mini Wonton Quiche
- Dinner: Spicy Cornbread with Coleslaw

Day 4:

- Breakfast: Bannock (Luskinikn)
- Lunch: Yogurt Feta Vegetable Dip with Crackers
- Dinner: Sour Cream with Cucumbers

Day 5:

- Breakfast: Fresh Fruit Cranberry Dip
- Lunch: A Slew Of Summer Fruits
- Dinner: Tortilla Chips with Sweet and Spicy Sauce

Day 6:

- Breakfast: Popcorn for a Special Day
- Lunch: Parfait With Pears And Almonds
- Dinner: Nutty Berry Parfait with Crab Dip

Day 7:

- Breakfast: Sweet & Sour Meatballs
- Lunch: Soup with Sour Cherries from Hungary
- Dinner: Spicy Cornbread with Coleslaw

<u>**Week 2:**</u>

Day 8:

- Breakfast: Bannock (Luskinikn)
- Lunch: Fresh Fruit Cranberry Dip
- Dinner: Chickpeas (Roasted) with Herbed Biscuits

Day 9:

- Breakfast: Bars of Granola
- Lunch: Yogurt Feta Vegetable Dip with Crackers
- Dinner: Sour Cream with Cucumbers

Day 10:
- Breakfast: Popcorn for a Special Day
- Lunch: A Slew Of Summer Fruits
- Dinner: Parfait With Pears And Almonds

Day 11:
- Breakfast: Almond Cookies from China
- Lunch: Delicious Deviled Eggs
- Dinner: Coleslaw with Cream with Crostini

Day 12:
- Breakfast: Lemon Sunburst Bars
- Lunch: Bites of Carrot Cake
- Dinner: Nutty Berry Parfait with Crab Dip

Day 13:
- Breakfast: Protein Bars with a Sweet and Nutty Flavor
- Lunch: Snack Combination with Delicious Ghanouj
- Dinner: Tuna Relish with Pizza

Day 14:
- Breakfast: Sweet & Sour Meatballs
- Lunch: Soup with Sour Cherries from Hungary
- Dinner: Spicy Cornbread with Coleslaw

For The Ebook Version, Scan The Code To Download

FOR ALL THE BOOKS WRITTEN BY THE AUTHOR SCAN HERE

www.ingramcontent.com/pod-product-compliance
Lightning Source LLC
Chambersburg PA
CBHW070854260726

48661CB00004B/1394